The Business of Personal Training

Helping Clients Achieve their Fitness Goals

Emerson Reagan

Introduction

In today's fast-paced and image-conscious world, the pursuit of fitness has become a universal aspiration. People of all ages and backgrounds are striving to achieve their desired level of health and physicality. And in the midst of this fitness revolution stands a crucial figure - the personal trainer.

The business of personal training has evolved far beyond simply guiding clients through workout routines. It has become a transformative force that empowers individuals to unleash their inner potential, break through limitations, and achieve their fitness goals. From shedding unwanted pounds to sculpting lean muscle, personal trainers have assumed the mantle of true agents of change.

But what exactly does it take to thrive in the world of personal training? How can one harness their passion for fitness and turn it into a successful and fulfilling career? This is a journey that encompasses not only a deep understanding of exercise science and nutrition but also the art of motivation, empathy, and enduring personal connections.

Through this compelling exploration, we will delve into the multidimensional world of personal training, uncovering its essential elements, and equipping you with the tools and insights necessary to make a substantial impact in the lives of your clients. From designing tailored fitness programs to effectively communicating with clients, from embracing technology to building a thriving business, we will leave no stone unturned in our quest to uncover the secrets of success in this booming industry.

Join us as we embark on this exhilarating journey, one that transcends the realms of physical exercise and plunges deep into the boundless potential of human transformation. Discover how to unlock the true power of personal training, helping clients become the very best versions of themselves, and making a lasting impact in their lives.

Are you ready to become a catalyst for change? Strap on your training shoes, because a world of opportunity awaits. Welcome to the fascinating realm of "The Business of Personal Training: Helping Clients Achieve their Fitness

Chapter one

Introduction to Personal Training

1.1 What is Personal Training?

Personal training is a specialized fitness profession that focuses on helping individuals achieve their health and fitness goals through personalized exercise and training programs. It involves a one-on-one approach, where a qualified personal trainer works closely with a client, tailoring workouts, providing guidance, and offering ongoing support to ensure optimal progress and results.

Unlike group fitness classes or generic workout routines, personal training takes into account the unique needs, abilities, and goals of each individual. The trainer evaluates the client's current fitness level, conducts assessments, and engages in open communication to understand their aspirations and limitations. This personalized approach allows the trainer to design a program that addresses the specific needs of the client, taking into consideration their fitness goals, preferences, and any existing medical conditions or injuries.

A personal trainer wears multiple hats throughout the journey of their clients. They are motivators, educators, and cheerleaders, offering constant encouragement and accountability. They provide continuous feedback and adjustment to ensure that the client is progressing effectively and safely toward their desired outcome.

Personal training is not limited to working with only those seeking weight loss or muscle gain. It caters to a wide range of fitness objectives, including improving cardiovascular health, increasing flexibility, enhancing sports performance, rehabilitating from injury, and reducing stress. With the clients' goals at the forefront, trainers employ a variety of training techniques, such as strength training, cardiovascular exercises, functional movements, and flexibility training, to create a well-rounded and balanced fitness routine.

In addition to the physical aspects of training, personal trainers also play a vital role in educating clients about proper nutrition, healthy lifestyle habits, and overall wellness. They provide guidance on dietary choices, portion control, and meal planning, which are crucial factors in achieving sustainable fitness results.

To become a personal trainer, individuals typically pursue specialized certifications and education in exercise science, anatomy, physiology, and various training methodologies. This knowledge equips trainers to navigate the complexities of the human body, enabling them to design programs that are both effective and safe.

Personal training has gained significant popularity in recent years, as individuals recognize the value of personalized attention and guidance in achieving their fitness goals. The personal trainer-client relationship goes beyond a simple fitness instructor-client transaction. It is a partnership built on trust, empathy, and dedication, with the ultimate aim of transforming lives and empowering individuals to reach their full potential.

1.2 Importance of Personal Training in Fitness Industry

Personal training plays a vital role in the ever-growing fitness industry. As more and more individuals recognize the importance of leading a healthy lifestyle and achieving their fitness goals, the demand for expert guidance and personalized training has skyrocketed. Below, we explore the key reasons why personal training is crucial in the fitness industry:

1. Customized Approach:

One of the standout benefits of personal training is the ability to tailor fitness programs to the specific needs and goals of each individual. No two people are the same, and what works for one person may not work for another. Personal trainers are adept at assessing clients' unique requirements, taking into account factors such as their physical abilities, medical history, lifestyle constraints, and preferences. They then design personalized workout routines that optimize results, minimize risk of injury, and provide the most effective path to achieving individual goals.

2. Motivation and Accountability:

Motivation is a key factor in maintaining a consistent exercise routine, but it can be challenging to stay motivated on your own. Personal trainers act as steadfast motivators, providing encouragement, guidance, and support throughout the fitness journey. They hold clients accountable for their actions, ensuring that they adhere to their exercise regimens and make progress toward their goals. This built-in accountability significantly increases the likelihood of clients staying committed to their fitness programs for the long term.

3. Proper Technique and Injury Prevention:

Practising proper exercise techniques is essential for maximizing results and minimizing the risk of injury. Personal trainers have extensive knowledge and experience in teaching correct form and execution for various exercises. They closely observe clients during workouts, providing immediate feedback and making necessary adjustments to ensure that exercises are performed safely and effectively. This reduces the likelihood of injuries caused by incorrect technique or overexertion.

4. Maximizing Efficiency and Results:

Time is a valuable resource for many individuals, and personal training helps clients make the most of their workout sessions. Trainers design efficient and effective workout routines that optimize the use of time and target specific fitness goals. Rather than aimlessly wandering through the gym or following generic exercise plans, clients benefit from structured, purposeful workouts that yield better results within a shorter duration.

5. Adapting to Individual Needs:

Personal training is particularly beneficial for individuals with specific needs or conditions. Whether a client is recovering from an injury, managing a chronic illness, or dealing with physical limitations, personal trainers can adapt workouts to accommodate these unique circumstances. They have the knowledge and skills to adjust exercises, incorporate modifications, and work in sync with healthcare professionals to ensure safe and effective training practices.

6. Education and Empowerment:

Beyond guiding clients through workouts, personal trainers empower individuals with knowledge and education about fitness, nutrition, and overall wellness. They provide valuable information on proper exercise techniques, effective training methods, and the science behind fitness. This enables clients to make informed decisions and empowers them to take control of their own health and well-being even outside of training sessions.

7. Long-term Lifestyle Changes:

Personal training goes beyond simply achieving short-term fitness goals. It aims to instil long-lasting lifestyle changes and habits that promote overall health and well-being. Trainers focus not only on exercise, but also on nutrition, stress management, and other lifestyle factors that impact fitness. By helping clients adopt sustainable habits and routines, personal trainers play a pivotal role in facilitating lasting positive change.

Chapter two
Becoming a Personal Trainer

2.1 Qualifications and Credentials

The field of personal training requires individuals to possess a strong knowledge base, specialized skills, and appropriate certifications to effectively guide clients on their fitness journeys. In the business of personal training, education and credentials are vital for credibility and trust. Below, we outline the key qualifications and credentials that aspiring personal trainers should consider obtaining:

1. Accredited Personal Training Certification:

The first step towards becoming a personal trainer is obtaining an accredited certification. There are numerous organizations that offer certifications, such as the American Council on Exercise (ACE), the National Academy of Sports Medicine (NASM), and the International Sports Sciences Association (ISSA). These certifications provide in-depth knowledge of exercise science, anatomy, physiology, program design, and instruction techniques. They typically require passing an exam that tests both theoretical knowledge and practical application.

2. Fitness Education and Academic Degrees:

While not mandatory, acquiring a higher education degree in a related field can enhance a personal trainer's knowledge and credibility. Pursuing a degree in exercise science, kinesiology, sports science, or a related discipline provides a comprehensive understanding of human anatomy, biomechanics, exercise physiology, and nutrition. Additionally, these programs often include practical experiences, internships, and research opportunities that further enrich a personal trainer's skill set.

3. Specialty Certifications:

Specialty certifications allow personal trainers to expand their expertise in specific areas and cater to a broader range of client needs. Some common speciality certifications include:

- Strength and Conditioning: Training athletes and enhancing sports performance.

- Corrective Exercise: Working with clients recovering from injuries, addressing muscular imbalances, and improving movement patterns.

- Weight Management: Providing specialized guidance on nutrition, weight loss, and body composition.

- Youth Fitness: Catering to the unique needs of children and teenagers, ensuring safe and effective workouts.

- Senior Fitness: Designing exercise programs specifically for older adults, considering age-related limitations and health concerns.

Obtaining specialty certifications demonstrates a personal trainer's commitment to continuous learning and their ability to meet the diverse needs of clients.

4. CPR and First Aid Certification:

As personal trainers are responsible for their clients' safety during workouts, possessing current certification in cardiopulmonary resuscitation (CPR) and first aid is fundamental. This certification ensures trainers are equipped with the necessary skills to respond effectively in case of emergencies or accidents that may occur during training sessions.

5. Continuing Education:

The fitness industry is constantly evolving, with new research, techniques, and training methodologies emerging regularly. Personal trainers should prioritize continuing education to stay up-to-date with the latest industry trends and advancements. Engaging in seminars, workshops, conferences, and online courses not only enhances knowledge but also serves as a testimony to a personal trainer's commitment to ongoing professional development.

6. Liability Insurance:

While not a qualification or certification, obtaining liability insurance is crucial for personal trainers. This insurance protects trainers from potential lawsuits arising from accidents, injuries, or claims associated with their services.

It helps trainers operate responsibly and provides a safety net in case unfortunate incidents occur.

2.2 Skills and Qualities of a Successful Personal Trainer

Becoming a successful personal trainer requires more than just technical knowledge or certifications. It also requires certain soft skills and qualities that allow trainers to connect with clients, provide effective coaching, and foster long-lasting relationships. Here are some key skills and qualities that successful personal trainers possess:

1. Communication:

The ability to communicate effectively is essential for a personal trainer. Trainers must be able to explain complex exercise science and fitness concepts to clients in an understandable way, ask questions to understand clients' needs and goals, listen actively to clients, and provide clear feedback and instruction. Possessing excellent communication skills helps trainers build trust, establish rapport, and foster positive client relationships.

2. Empathy and Understanding:

Personal trainers need to connect with clients on a personal level to understand their concerns, challenges, and goals. Empathy and understanding involve recognizing and respecting clients' individual differences, acknowledging their successes and struggles, and providing support and motivation throughout their fitness journey. Trainers who show empathy and understanding create a supportive and non-judgmental environment that helps clients feel comfortable, motivated, and inspired.

3. Patience:

Progress in fitness takes time, and personal trainers must have patience when working with clients. Successful trainers understand that results don't happen overnight, and constant motivation and encouragement are needed to keep clients on track. They also recognize that everyone has different abilities and that workouts need to be customized and adaptive to accommodate clients' needs and limitations. Personal trainers who possess patience are better equipped to sustain long-term relationships with clients, even in the face of setbacks and obstacles.

4. Adaptability:

Personal trainers must be adaptable to cater to clients' unique needs and goals. They must be able to adjust exercise programs based on clients' abilities and limitations, adapt to clients' schedules and preferences, and implement alternative training strategies when necessary. Personal trainers who display adaptability create positive experiences for clients, helping them stay engaged and motivated throughout the fitness journey.

5. Time Management and Organization:

Personal trainers work with clients with differing schedules and availability, and must be able to manage their time effectively to maintain a prosperous business. Successful personal trainers can organize their workday effectively, prioritize tasks, and schedule client sessions with ease. They know how to make the most of their time, maintain professionalism and punctuality, and ensure that clients receive the attention and personalized care they deserve.

6. Enthusiasm and Passion:

Personal trainers who love what they do are more likely to be successful at it. Trainers who possess enthusiasm and passion for fitness and helping others achieve their goals are more likely to create an environment that is supportive and energizing. They are motivated to stay current with industry trends, adopt new techniques, and seek out best practices. Personal trainers who are enthusiastic and passionate about their work create memorable experiences for their clients and inspire them to push past their limits.

2.3 Career Options and Opportunities

Becoming a personal trainer can lead to a rewarding and fulfilling career path with numerous opportunities for growth and development. From working in a gym or fitness studio to starting a business as an entrepreneur, personal trainers have various options to choose from. Here are some career options and opportunities available for personal trainers:

1. Working in a Gym or Fitness Studio:

The most common career path for personal trainers is working in a gym or fitness studio. Gyms and fitness studios provide personal trainers with a steady stream of clients and offer a range of equipment and resources to help trainers excel in their work. Personal trainers working in a gym or studio can expect to receive a stable income and benefits, such as paid time off, health insurance, and retirement plans.

2. Starting a Personal Training Business:

Becoming an entrepreneur and starting a personal training business is another option for personal trainers. Starting a personal training business allows trainers to be their own boss, set their own schedule, and create their own unique brand. However, starting a business requires a lot of work and dedication, including the establishment of a client base, managing finances, and marketing strategies.

3. Online Personal Training:

The advancements in digital technologies have created new opportunities for personal trainers. Online personal training provides trainers with the ability to reach a broader audience beyond their geographical location. Personal trainers can use platforms such as social media, online fitness apps, and websites to reach clients and provide virtual coaching and training services. Online personal training offers a flexible schedule and more autonomy over personal training services.

4. Corporate Fitness:

Corporate fitness is a growing field that provides opportunities for personal trainers to work with corporate clients and help them maintain healthy lifestyles. Corporate fitness trainers design fitness programs that fit around their client's work schedules and offer group training sessions.

Personal trainers working in corporate fitness can expect to receive competitive salaries and benefits.

5. Group Fitness Instruction:

For personal trainers who enjoy leading group fitness classes, there is an opportunity to teach group fitness. This role requires a certification in group fitness instruction and requires the ability to lead and motivate a group of individuals with varying levels of fitness.

6. Specialized Personal Training:

Specialized personal training allows personal trainers to provide specialized services to a specific population of clients. Personal trainers who specialize in areas such as post-rehabilitation, youth training, senior fitness, and sports performance can find opportunities for employment in sports training facilities, rehabilitation centers, and hospitals.

7. Fitness Journalism and Writing:

For personal trainers who enjoy writing about health and fitness, a career in fitness journalism and writing is an option. Fitness journalists work with different publications, websites, and all forms of digital content creation that require knowledge in fitness and health.

Chapter three
Understanding Clients

3.1 Assessing the Fitness Needs of Clients

Assessing the fitness needs of clients is a crucial step in the personal training process. It allows personal trainers to gain a comprehensive understanding of their clients' goals, abilities, and limitations. By conducting thorough assessments, trainers can tailor their programs to meet the specific needs of each client. Here are some key considerations and methods for assessing the fitness needs of clients:

1. Initial Consultation:

The initial consultation is the first step in assessing the fitness needs of clients. During this meeting, personal trainers gather information about clients' goals, medical history, exercise preferences, and lifestyle factors. It is important to ask open-ended questions and actively listen to clients' responses to gain a deeper understanding of their motivations and expectations.

2. Health and Fitness Questionnaires:
Health and fitness questionnaires are valuable tools for gathering comprehensive information about clients' medical history, previous exercise experience, current lifestyle habits, and any existing injuries or health conditions. These questionnaires help trainers identify any potential risks or limitations that may affect the exercise program design.

3. Physical Fitness Assessments:
Performing physical fitness assessments allows personal trainers to gauge clients' current fitness levels and identify

areas that need improvement. Common assessments include body composition analysis, cardiovascular fitness testing, muscular strength and endurance evaluation, flexibility testing, and functional movement screening. These assessments provide a baseline measurement of clients' abilities and serve as a reference point to track progress over time.

4. Functional Movement Screening:

Functional movement screening is a valuable assessment tool that evaluates clients' movement patterns and identifies any imbalances, asymmetries, or limitations. By observing how clients move, trainers can detect any biomechanical issues that may contribute to pain, injury, or decreased performance. Functional movement screening helps trainers develop exercise programs that address specific movement deficiencies and promote optimal performance.

5. Goal Setting:

Setting clear and realistic goals is an essential part of understanding clients' fitness needs. Personal trainers work closely with clients to define both short-term and long-term goals that are specific, measurable, achievable, relevant, and time-bound (SMART goals). Goals should align with clients' desires and be challenging yet attainable to maintain their motivation and commitment.

6. Communication and Client Feedback:

Effective communication and regular feedback loops are crucial for understanding clients' evolving fitness needs. Trainers should encourage open and honest communication, listen attentively to clients' questions and concerns, and proactively seek feedback on their training experience. Regular check-ins provide an opportunity to fine-tune the exercise program, address any issues or challenges, and celebrate milestones.

7. Re-assessments:

Re-assessments are essential to track progress and adapt the exercise program as clients' fitness levels improve. Regularly reviewing and updating assessments help personal trainers measure clients' achievements, identify any plateaus or setbacks, and make appropriate adjustments to the training program to keep clients challenged and engaged.

3.2 Goal Setting and Planning

Goal setting is a critical component of personal training as it helps personal trainers and clients establish a clear direction and purpose for their fitness journey. By understanding clients' goals and creating a structured plan, trainers can effectively guide their clients towards achieving their desired outcomes. Here are some key considerations and strategies for goal setting and planning with clients:

1. Establish Clear Goals:

The first step in goal setting is to establish clear and specific goals with clients. This involves understanding what clients want to achieve, whether it's weight loss, muscle gain, improved cardiovascular fitness, or increased flexibility. Trainers should help clients define their goals in measurable terms, such as losing a certain number of pounds or being able to run a specific distance within a given time frame. Clear goals provide a benchmark to track progress and maintain motivation.

2. Assess Current Fitness Levels:

Before creating a plan, it is essential to assess clients' current fitness levels. This assessment helps trainers gauge clients' starting point and identify any areas that require improvement. By understanding clients' strengths and weaknesses, trainers can design appropriate exercise programs that address individual needs and promote steady progress.

3. Break Goals into Actionable Steps:

Once goals are established, trainers should break them down into smaller, actionable steps. Setting milestone goals along the way helps clients stay motivated and focused. For example, if a client's ultimate goal is to complete a half-marathon, the trainer can set intermediate goals such as running a 5K and 10K race. Breaking down goals into manageable steps creates a sense of accomplishment and encourages continued effort.

4. Create a Tailored Exercise Program:

Based on clients' goals and current fitness levels, trainers should develop a tailored exercise program. The program should include a variety of exercises that target specific goals, such as strength training, cardiovascular training, flexibility training, and functional movements. The program should also take into account clients' preferences, time constraints, and any physical limitations or injuries to ensure safety and sustainability.

5. Incorporate SMART Goals:

The use of SMART goals (Specific, Measurable, Achievable, Relevant, Time-bound) can enhance the effectiveness of goal setting. Trainers should help clients set goals that are specific and clearly defined, measurable to track progress, achievable within clients' capabilities, relevant to their overall fitness objectives, and time-bound with a specific timeline for achievement. SMART goals provide a framework for creating realistic and attainable targets.

6. Adaptability and Flexibility:

It is important to recognize that goals and plans may need to be adjusted over time as clients progress or encounter unexpected challenges. Trainers should regularly review and update goals based on clients' achievements, feedback, and changing circumstances. The ability to adapt and modify the exercise program ensures that it remains challenging and aligned with clients' evolving needs.

7. Provide Support and Accountability:

Establishing a supportive and accountable relationship with clients is crucial for goal achievement. Trainers should provide ongoing guidance, encouragement, and feedback to help clients stay motivated and on track. Regular check-ins, progress tracking, and open communication create a sense of accountability and ensure that clients remain committed to their goals.

8. Celebrate Milestones:

Recognizing and celebrating clients' milestones and achievements is essential for maintaining motivation and providing positive reinforcement. Personal trainers should acknowledge and celebrate progress, whether it's reaching a specific weight-loss milestone, improving strength, or completing a challenging workout. Celebrating milestones reinforces clients' commitment and boosts their confidence in their ability to achieve their ultimate goals.

3.3 Client Communication and Motivation Techniques

Effective client communication and motivation techniques are essential for personal trainers to establish strong relationships with their clients and help them achieve their fitness goals. By understanding clients' needs, preferences, and motivations, trainers can tailor their coaching style and strategies to maximize engagement and adherence to the exercise program. Here are some key considerations and techniques for client communication and motivation in the context of personal training:

1. Active Listening:

Active listening is a fundamental skill that personal trainers should possess to understand their clients' needs and concerns. This involves giving full attention to clients, asking probing questions to clarify information, and responding empathetically. By actively listening, trainers can gain valuable insights into clients' motivations, challenges, and personal preferences, which can inform the exercise program and enhance client satisfaction.

2. Building Rapport and Trust:

Developing rapport and trust is crucial for effective communication and motivation. Trainers should create a friendly and supportive environment where clients feel comfortable sharing their thoughts and concerns. Building a strong rapport involves demonstrating genuine interest, displaying empathy, and maintaining confidentiality. Clients who trust and feel understood by their trainers are more likely to stay engaged and motivated throughout their fitness journey.

3. Understanding Motivational Factors:

Personal trainers should strive to understand the motivational factors that drive their clients. Motivation can vary from person to person, whether it be improving overall health, achieving a specific aesthetic appearance, or excelling in a particular sport. By understanding clients' motivations, trainers can tailor their coaching techniques and program design to align with clients' goals, making the experience more meaningful and engaging.

4. Setting Realistic Expectations:

To keep clients motivated, it is important to set realistic expectations from the beginning. Personal trainers should help clients understand that fitness goals take time and consistent effort to achieve. By setting achievable milestones and celebrating progress along the way, trainers can keep clients motivated and encouraged to continue their fitness journey.

5. Communication Channels:

Personal trainers should consider clients' preferred communication channels and adapt their communication methods accordingly. Some clients may prefer face-to-face interactions, while others may prefer email, text messages, or phone calls. Understanding clients' communication preferences allows trainers to establish efficient and effective channels that support ongoing communication and feedback.

6. Positive Reinforcement:

Providing positive reinforcement is a powerful technique to motivate clients. Recognizing and praising clients' efforts, milestones achieved, and improvements made fosters a sense of accomplishment and boosts confidence. Regularly acknowledging clients' progress reinforces their commitment and helps them stay motivated throughout their fitness journey.

7. Goal Recap and Progress Updates:

Regularly recapping goals and providing progress updates is instrumental in maintaining motivation. Trainers should remind clients of their goals and show them how far they have come. Progress updates can include measurements, performance improvements, or simply reminding clients of the positive changes they have experienced. Seeing tangible evidence of progress can empower clients and motivate them to push further.

8. Continuous Education and Support:

Providing ongoing education and support is vital for keeping clients engaged and motivated. Trainers should keep clients informed about the science behind the exercises, health benefits, and proper nutrition. Additionally, offering educational resources such as articles, videos, or workshops can further empower clients on their fitness journey. Continuous support, whether it be through regular check-ins, answering questions promptly, or providing additional resources, demonstrates the trainer's commitment to their clients' success.

9. Individualized Coaching:

Personal trainers should recognize that each client is unique and requires individualized coaching. While some clients may respond well to high-intensity workouts, others may prefer a more leisurely pace. Trainers must adapt their coaching style and exercise program to accommodate individual needs, preferences, and abilities. By tailoring the training experience to clients' specific requirements, trainers can maximize client satisfaction and motivation.

10. Goal Adjustments and New Challenges:

As clients progress and achieve their initial goals, it is important to reassess and establish new challenges.

Trainers should help clients set new goals that are slightly more ambitious, ensuring continued growth and motivation. By regularly adjusting goals and introducing new challenges, trainers keep clients engaged and excited about their fitness journey.

Chapter four

Designing Effective Fitness Programs

4.1 Principles of Fitness Training

Designing effective fitness programs is a crucial aspect of personal training, as it lays the foundation for clients to achieve their goals and improve their overall health and wellness. By following the principles of fitness training, personal trainers can create tailored programs that are safe, progressive, and yield optimal results. Here are some key principles to consider when designing fitness programs for clients:

1. Individualization:

One of the fundamental principles of fitness training is individualization. Personal trainers should take into account clients' unique needs, goals, preferences, and physical capabilities when designing their fitness programs. Each client has different starting points, fitness levels, and limitations that must be considered to create a program that is both challenging and achievable. By tailoring programs to individual needs, trainers can maximize client engagement and overall success.

2. Specificity:

The principle of specificity emphasizes that the exercise program should align with clients' goals and desired outcomes. Different exercises and training modalities produce specific adaptations in the body. For example, someone focused on strength training will have a different program than someone targeting weight loss or improving cardiovascular endurance. Personal trainers must understand clients' goals and design programs that prioritize the specific adaptations required to achieve those goals.

3. Progressive Overload:

Progressive overload is the gradual increase in intensity, duration, or frequency of exercise over time. It is an essential principle for continual improvement and achieving desired outcomes. Personal trainers should progressively challenge clients' bodies by increasing the demands placed on their muscles, cardiovascular system, or flexibility. By progressively overloading the body, trainers can stimulate adaptation and ensure ongoing progress.

4. Variation and Periodization:

Variation and periodization refer to systematically altering the training variables, such as exercise selection, intensity, volume, and rest intervals. Varying the workouts helps prevent plateaus, reduces the risk of overuse injuries, and keeps clients motivated and engaged. Periodization involves systematically manipulating training variables over a specific timeframe, typically divided into phases such as hypertrophy, strength, power, and recovery. By incorporating variation and periodization, trainers can optimize clients' progress and overall performance.

5. Safety and Injury Prevention:

Personal trainers have a responsibility to prioritize client safety and prevent injuries. This involves proper exercise technique instruction, suitable exercise selection, appropriate progression, and ensuring clients are adequately warmed up and cooled down. Trainers should have a thorough understanding of biomechanics and exercise physiology to identify and correct faulty movement patterns or risky exercises. By prioritizing safety, trainers can create an environment that fosters long-term success and minimizes the risk of injury.

6. Individual Recovery and Rest:

Rest and recovery are vital components of an effective fitness program. Personal trainers should emphasize the importance of incorporating adequate rest periods and recovery strategies into clients' routines. This includes incorporating rest days, utilizing different training modalities (such as active recovery or mobility work), and encouraging clients to prioritize sleep and nutrition. By allowing the body to recover and adapt, trainers can optimize performance and reduce the risk of overtraining and burnout.

7. Adherence and Sustainability:

An effective fitness program should be designed with the client's long-term adherence and sustainability in mind. Personal trainers should consider clients' preferences, lifestyle, and time constraints when creating their programs. By designing programs that fit seamlessly into clients' lives, trainers can enhance adherence and promote long-term success. Additionally, trainers should educate clients on the importance of finding activities they enjoy to make exercise more enjoyable and sustainable in the long run.

8. Regular Assessment and Modifications:

Fitness programs should not be static, but rather dynamic and adaptable to clients' progress and changing needs. Regular assessment of clients' performance, goals, and feedback allows trainers to make appropriate modifications to the program. By continually assessing and adjusting the program, trainers can ensure it remains challenging, aligned with clients' goals, and responsive to their evolving capabilities.

9. Education and Empowerment:

Personal trainers have a responsibility to educate and empower their clients. This involves providing explanations and demonstrations of exercises, educating clients on the principles behind the program, and explaining the benefits of each component. Trainers should teach clients how to track progress, adjust intensity, and make informed decisions about their exercise and lifestyle choices. By empowering clients with knowledge, trainers increase their ownership and commitment to their fitness journey.

4.2 Program Design for Different Fitness Goals (Weight Loss, Muscle Building, Endurance, etc.)

Designing effective fitness programs involves tailoring the program to clients' specific goals. Different fitness goals require different approaches and training modalities to achieve optimal results. Whether the goal is weight loss, muscle building, endurance improvement, or a combination of these, personal trainers need to understand the unique requirements of each goal and design programs accordingly. Here are some key considerations for program design based on different fitness goals:

1. Weight Loss:

Weight loss is a common goal for many individuals seeking personal training. To create an effective program for weight loss, personal trainers should focus on a combination of cardiovascular exercise, strength training, and proper nutrition. Cardiovascular activities such as running, cycling, or HIIT workouts help burn calories and promote fat loss. Strength training is crucial to preserve muscle mass and boost metabolism. Additionally, trainers should emphasize creating a caloric deficit through proper nutrition and include strategies to increase clients' overall daily activity level.

2. Muscle Building:

For clients looking to build muscle mass, personal trainers should emphasize resistance training and progressive overload. The program should focus on compound exercises that target major muscle groups, such as squats, deadlifts, bench press, and rows. Trainers should incorporate a variety of resistance training methods, including free weights, machines, and bodyweight exercises, to stimulate muscle growth. Progressive overload, achieved through increasing weight, reps, sets, or decreasing rest intervals, is necessary for continuous muscle adaptation and growth. Adequate protein intake and proper recovery strategies are also essential for muscle building.

3. Endurance Improvement:

Clients seeking to improve their endurance, whether for running, cycling, or other endurance-based activities, require programs that prioritize cardiovascular training and muscular endurance. Trainers should incorporate cardiovascular exercises such as running, cycling, swimming, or rowing to improve the clients' cardiovascular capacity. High-intensity interval training (HIIT) is particularly effective for improving endurance by alternating between periods of intense effort and recovery. Additionally, muscular endurance exercises, such as bodyweight circuits or light resistance training with higher repetitions, help enhance the muscles' ability to sustain repeated contractions.

4. Strength and Power:

Clients aiming to improve their overall strength and power require programs that emphasize heavy resistance training, explosive movements, and plyometrics. Personal trainers should focus on compound exercises using challenging weights and low repetitions to build maximum strength. Power training, involving explosive movements like plyometrics, medicine ball throws, or Olympic lifts, helps develop quick and powerful movements. Trainers should also incorporate exercises that target specific muscle groups or movements that are relevant to the client's goals, such as jumping or sprinting.

5. Flexibility and Mobility:

Flexibility and mobility are essential for overall joint health, injury prevention, and functional movement. Personal trainers should incorporate stretching exercises, dynamic warm-ups, and mobility drills into the program to improve clients' range of motion and joint mobility. Static stretching should be performed both during warm-ups and as a cool-down to enhance flexibility. Additionally, trainers should educate clients on the importance of incorporating regular stretching and mobility exercises into their daily routines to maintain and improve overall flexibility.

6. Combination Goals:

Many clients have a combination of goals and may want to focus on multiple aspects, such as weight loss and muscle building or strength and endurance. Personal trainers should design programs that combine elements of each goal while maintaining a balanced approach. This may involve alternating between strength training and cardiovascular exercises, incorporating circuit training or metabolic conditioning workouts, or periodizing the training program to prioritize different goals in specific phases.

Trainers should also ensure proper nutrition and recovery strategies align with the clients' combined goals.

4.3 Nutrition and Diet Considerations in Fitness Programs

When designing effective fitness programs, it is essential to consider nutrition and diet as crucial components. Proper nutrition plays a vital role in achieving fitness goals, whether it is weight loss, muscle building, or endurance improvement. Personal trainers should educate clients on the importance of nutrition and help them make informed choices to support their fitness journey. Here are some key considerations for nutrition and diet in fitness programs:

1. Energy Balance:

Energy balance is the relationship between the calories consumed through food and the calories expended through physical activity. To achieve weight-related fitness goals, such as weight loss or muscle gain, it is important to create an appropriate energy balance. Personal trainers should assess clients' current energy intake and expenditure and make necessary adjustments. For weight loss, creating a calorie deficit by consuming fewer calories than expended is essential, while for muscle building, a calorie surplus may be required.

2. Macronutrient Distribution:

Macronutrients, including carbohydrates, proteins, and fats, are essential for overall health and optimal performance. The distribution of these macronutrients should align with clients' goals. For example, weight loss programs may prioritize a higher protein intake to support muscle preservation and appetite control. Muscle building programs require adequate protein for muscle repair and synthesis. Endurance training programs often emphasize proper carbohydrate intake to fuel performance. Personal trainers should educate clients on the importance of each macronutrient and help them establish an appropriate distribution within their diet.

3. Meal Timing and Frequency:

Personal trainers should provide guidance on meal timing and frequency to optimize clients' energy levels and performance. The timing of meals and snacks before and after workouts can significantly impact energy availability, recovery, and muscle synthesis. Trainers may recommend pre-workout meals or snacks that provide a combination of carbohydrates and protein for sustained energy. Post-workout nutrition should focus on replenishing glycogen stores and promoting muscle repair and recovery. Additionally, trainers can discuss the benefits of regular meals and snacks throughout the day to maintain stable blood sugar levels and avoid excessive hunger.

4. Hydration:

Hydration is a critical aspect of fitness programs as proper fluid intake is essential for performance and overall health. Personal trainers should educate clients on the importance of hydration and provide guidelines for fluid intake before, during, and after workouts. Trainers can assess clients' fluid needs based on factors like body weight, activity level, and environmental conditions. Adequate hydration can support optimal cognitive function, temperature regulation, and muscle contractions during exercise.

5. Nutrient Timing and Supplements:

Nutrient timing refers to the strategic consumption of nutrients before, during, and after exercise to optimize performance, recovery, and adaptation. Personal trainers should educate clients on the benefits of proper nutrient timing and discuss strategies such as consuming carbohydrates and protein before workouts or using recovery shakes post-workout. Additionally, trainers can provide information on supplements that may benefit clients' specific goals, such as whey protein, creatine, or omega-3 fatty acids. However, trainers should emphasize that whole foods should always be the primary source of nutrients, and supplementation should be used with caution and under professional guidance.

6. Individual Dietary Considerations:

Personal trainers should take into account clients' individual dietary considerations, preferences, and restrictions when designing fitness programs. Some clients may have specific dietary restrictions, allergies, or cultural preferences that need to be addressed. By understanding clients' unique needs, trainers can provide appropriate alternatives and recommendations to ensure the program is sustainable and enjoyable.

7. Education and Behavior Change:

Personal trainers have an important role in educating clients about nutrition and facilitating behaviour change. Trainers should provide clients with evidence-based information on nutrition and emphasize the importance of creating sustainable and realistic dietary habits. They can assist clients in setting nutrition-related goals, monitoring progress, and making necessary adjustments. Trainers can also recommend reliable resources, such as registered dietitians or nutritionists, for clients who may require more specialized guidance.

8. Continual Support and Accountability:

Support and accountability are essential for clients to adhere to their nutrition goals. Personal trainers can provide ongoing support by checking in with clients regularly, providing feedback on food choices, and helping troubleshoot any challenges or obstacles they may face. Trainers can also encourage keeping a food diary or using nutrition tracking applications to promote awareness and accountability.

Chapter five

Exercise Techniques and Safety

5.1 Correct Form and Techniques for Various Exercises

Proper form and technique are crucial when performing exercises in a fitness program. Correct form not only ensures optimal results but also reduces the risk of injury. Personal trainers have a responsibility to educate clients on the proper form and technique for various exercises to promote safety and effectiveness. Here are some key considerations for correct form and techniques:

1. Exercise Instruction:

Personal trainers should provide clear and detailed instructions on how to perform each exercise correctly.

They should demonstrate the exercise themselves and explain the movement patterns, body positioning, and range of motion. Trainers should also emphasize the importance of starting with light weights or bodyweight exercises before progressing to heavier loads.

2. Body Alignment and Posture:

Proper body alignment and posture are essential for maintaining safety and maximizing the effectiveness of exercises. Trainers should guide clients on maintaining a neutral spine, engaging the core muscles, and proper joint alignment throughout each exercise. Emphasizing proper alignment reduces the risk of strains, overuse injuries, and chronic pain.

3. Breathing Technique:

Proper breathing technique is often overlooked but plays a significant role in exercise performance and safety.

Trainers should instruct clients on the appropriate breathing pattern for each exercise. For example, for strength exercises, clients should exhale during the exertion phase and inhale during the relaxation phase. Proper breathing supports stability, and oxygenation of muscles, and prevents excessive intra-abdominal pressure.

4. Range of Motion:

Correct range of motion (ROM) ensures that clients are activating the intended muscles and joints effectively. Personal trainers should demonstrate and educate clients on the appropriate ROM for each exercise. Ensuring a full range of motion helps improve flexibility, joint mobility, and muscle activation while minimizing the risk of muscle imbalances or overuse injuries.

5. Tempo and Speed:

Exercise tempo refers to the speed or rhythm at which an exercise is performed. Trainers should instruct clients on the appropriate tempo for each exercise, including eccentric (muscle lengthening), concentric (muscle shortening), and isometric (static) phases. Controlling tempo helps maintain proper form, enhances muscle control, and prevents momentum-based movements that can compromise safety and results.

6. Exercise Modifications and Progressions:

Personal trainers should be knowledgeable in exercise modifications and progressions to cater to clients' individual needs and abilities. Modifications may include using lighter weights, resistance bands, or modifying body positioning to accommodate injuries, limitations, or fitness levels. Progressions involve gradually increasing the intensity, complexity, or resistance of exercises as clients become more proficient. By providing appropriate modifications and progressions, trainers can ensure safety, prevent plateaus, and maintain client motivation.

7. Rest and Recovery:

Trainers should educate clients on the importance of rest and recovery in their exercise programs. Rest periods between sets or exercises allow for proper muscle recovery and prevent overexertion. Trainers should guide clients on the appropriate amount of rest based on the exercise intensity and individual fitness level.

8. Preventing Common Mistakes:

Personal trainers should be proactive in identifying and correcting common exercise mistakes that clients may make. Common mistakes include rounding the back, using excessive momentum, improper grip or foot placement, or performing exercises too quickly. By addressing and correcting these mistakes, trainers can prevent injuries and ensure clients are getting the most out of their workouts.

9. Safety Considerations:

Trainers should always prioritize safety when teaching exercises. This includes ensuring appropriate warm-up and cool-down, providing clear and stable surfaces for exercise, instructing proper use of equipment, and monitoring clients for signs of fatigue or discomfort. Personal trainers should be prepared to modify or adapt exercises to maintain safety, particularly for clients with specific health conditions or limitations.

10. Regular Form and Technique Assessment:

Assessing and reinforcing correct form and technique should be an ongoing process in personal training. Trainers should regularly observe clients' movements, provide feedback, and make necessary corrections. This continual assessment helps clients develop muscle memory, improve exercise efficiency, and prevent the development of bad habits.

5.2 Preventing and Handling Injuries

Injuries can occur during exercise, but with proper prevention strategies and knowledge of how to respond in case of injury, personal trainers can ensure the safety and well-being of their clients. Preventing injuries should be a priority in any fitness program, and personal trainers play a crucial role in educating clients on injury prevention techniques and knowing how to handle injuries should they occur. Here are some key considerations for preventing and handling injuries:

1. Pre-Exercise Assessment:

Before starting any exercise program, personal trainers should conduct a thorough assessment of their clients' health history, previous injuries, and any pre-existing conditions or limitations. This assessment helps identify potential risk factors and allows trainers to tailor the program to the individual's needs.

2. Proper Warm-up:

A proper warm-up is essential to prepare the body for exercise and minimize the risk of injury. Trainers should guide clients through dynamic movements, mobility exercises, and light cardiovascular activity to increase blood flow, raise body temperature, and activate the muscles. A warm-up should be specific to the exercises planned for the workout and gradually increase in intensity.

3. Correct Form and Technique:

Proper form and technique not only optimize exercise effectiveness but also play a significant role in injury prevention. Trainers should ensure that clients understand and perform exercises with correct form, focusing on maintaining proper posture, joint alignment, and range of motion. Regular monitoring and feedback from trainers can help correct any deviations and reduce the risk of injury.

4. Gradual Progression:

Progressing exercise intensity and difficulty gradually is crucial for preventing injuries. Trainers should employ progressive overload principles, increasing intensity, duration, or load incrementally to allow the body to adapt and minimize the risk of overuse injuries. Pushing clients too quickly can lead to strains, sprains, or stress fractures.

5. Cross-training and Variation:

Including a variety of exercises and incorporating cross-training techniques can reduce the risk of overuse injuries. Personal trainers should encourage clients to engage in different types of exercise, such as strength training, cardiovascular workouts, and flexibility/mobility exercises. This variation allows different muscle groups to be worked, reduces repetitive stress on specific areas, and promotes overall muscular balance.

6. Listen to the Body:

Trainers should emphasize the importance of listening to their bodies and recognizing warning signs during exercise. Encouraging clients to pay attention to pain, discomfort, or unusual sensations can prevent minor issues from developing into more severe injuries. Trainers should educate clients on the difference between muscle soreness and pain and advise them to seek medical attention for persistent or severe pain.

7. Nutrition and Hydration:

Proper nutrition and hydration play a significant role in injury prevention. Trainers should educate clients on the importance of balanced nutrition to support muscle recovery and repair. Adequate hydration ensures optimal muscle function, joint lubrication, and temperature regulation. Recommending a diet rich in essential nutrients and appropriate fluid intake promotes injury prevention and overall well-being.

8. Rest and Recovery:

Rest and recovery are essential components of any fitness program. Personal trainers should educate clients on the importance of rest days, proper sleep, and recovery techniques such as foam rolling or stretching. Overtraining and lack of recovery can lead to fatigue, decreased performance, and increased susceptibility to injuries.

9. Injury Response and First Aid:

In the event of an injury during a training session, personal trainers should be equipped with the knowledge of basic first aid response. This includes assessing the severity of the injury, applying appropriate first aid techniques (such as RICE: rest, ice, compression, elevation), and knowing when to seek medical attention. Trainers should prioritize the immediate well-being and safety of the client, ensuring they receive appropriate medical advice or care.

10. Rehabilitation and Referral:

If a client experiences an injury that requires rehabilitation, personal trainers should collaborate with healthcare professionals, such as physical therapists or sports medicine specialists. Trainers should facilitate communication between the client and the healthcare provider, providing relevant information on the nature of the injury and any modifications needed in the exercise program. This collaboration ensures a safe and effective path to recovery.

5.3 Ensuring Client Safety during Exercise Sessions

Ensuring client safety during exercise sessions is of the utmost importance for personal trainers. Creating a safe environment for clients not only minimizes the risk of injury but also establishes trust and builds a positive trainer-client relationship. Personal trainers need to take appropriate measures to ensure client safety during exercise sessions. Here are some key considerations for ensuring client safety:

1. Good Communication:

Clear communication between a personal trainer and a client is essential for ensuring client safety. Trainers should explain each exercise to the client, demonstrating proper form and technique. This ensures that the client understands the movement patterns, range of motion, and potential risks associated with each exercise. Trainers should also listen to clients' concerns, acknowledge their limitations, and modify exercises accordingly.

2. Proper Equipment and Environment:

A safe exercise environment should include properly maintained equipment, adequate space, and proper ventilation. Trainers should ensure that equipment is in good condition, free of any defects, and regularly sanitized. The exercise space should be well-lit, have appropriate flooring, and be free of obstacles. Proper ventilation ensures adequate air exchange, preventing overheating and improving overall client comfort.

3. Client Health Screening:

Before starting any exercise program, personal trainers should conduct health screenings to collect information on the client's health status. This includes medical history, current medications, and any physical limitations. This information helps trainers identify specific needs and limitations and modify exercises accordingly. If any underlying conditions are identified, trainers may also need to seek medical clearance from a healthcare provider.

4. Proper Warm-up and Cool-down:

A proper warm-up is essential to prevent injuries and prepare the body for exercise. Trainers should design a warm-up that is specific to the exercises planned, gradually increasing intensity to raise the body's temperature and increase blood flow. A cool-down is also important to allow the heart rate and breathing to return to normal and prevent dizziness or fainting. Trainers should devote adequate time to both warm-up and cool-down.

5. Gradual Progression:

Gradual progression in exercise intensity, duration, or load is necessary to prevent injuries and avoid overexertion. Trainers should monitor the client's response to exercise and modify the program as needed. Pushing clients too quickly can lead to strain, sprain, or stress fractures and should be avoided.

6. Client Feedback:

Trainers should encourage clients to provide feedback during exercise sessions. This includes monitoring fatigue, pain, or discomfort during exercise and communicating this information to the trainer. It also involves monitoring changes in mood, energy, and overall well-being. Trainers should be responsive to this feedback and modify the exercise program accordingly.

7. Proper Form and Technique:

Proper form and technique are essential for preventing injuries and ensuring exercise effectiveness. Trainers should teach clients the correct form and technique for each exercise, emphasizing maintaining proper posture, joint alignment, and range of motion. Clients should be monitored to ensure that they are performing exercises correctly and modifications made if necessary.

8. Proper Breathing Technique:

Proper breathing technique is often overlooked but is important for maintaining stability and preventing injuries. Clients should be instructed on appropriate breathing techniques for each exercise. This includes exhaling during the effort phase and inhaling during the relaxation phase. Trainers should monitor clients to ensure proper breathing technique is maintained.

9. Emergency Preparedness:

In the event of an emergency, trainers should have a plan in place. This includes knowing the location of first aid equipment, the procedure for calling emergency services, and guiding clients through appropriate first aid techniques. Trainers should be trained in CPR and have completed a first aid course to respond to emergencies.

10. Injury Prevention Education:

Educating clients on injury prevention techniques is crucial for maintaining client safety. Trainers should provide information on warming up, cool-down, appropriate equipment use, and progressive exercise overload, as well as monitoring feedback from clients. By educating clients on proper exercise techniques and injury prevention strategies, clients can feel confident and safe during exercise sessions.

Chapter six

Personal Training Tools and Technology

6.1 Importance of Technology in Personal Training

Technology has become an integral part of our lives, and the fitness industry is no exception. In the field of personal training, the use of technology has revolutionized the way trainers interact with clients, track progress, and provide personalized training programs. Personal training tools and technology have significantly enhanced the effectiveness and efficiency of personal training services. Here are some key reasons why technology is important in personal training:

1. Enhanced Communication:

Technology has greatly improved communication between personal trainers and clients. Trainers can use various communication platforms, such as email, messaging apps, or video calls, to stay in touch with clients outside of training sessions. This allows for easy and quick communication regarding progress updates, scheduling changes, or any questions that clients may have. It also helps build a stronger relationship between trainers and clients, resulting in more effective training.

2. Online Training Programs:

The integration of technology in personal training has made online training programs possible. This provides flexibility and convenience for both trainers and clients. Trainers can design and deliver comprehensive training programs through online platforms or mobile apps, allowing clients to access their workouts and training materials anytime, anywhere. Online training programs also enable trainers to reach a broader client base beyond their geographical location.

3. Individualized Training:

Personal training tools and technology allow trainers to provide highly individualized training programs. Fitness apps, wearables, and software can collect and analyze data on clients' activity levels, heart rate, sleep patterns, and more. Trainers can use this information to tailor workouts and track progress, ensuring that clients are working at an appropriate intensity and achieving optimal results. This level of personalization boosts client motivation and helps them reach their goals faster.

4. Performance Tracking:

Technology provides trainers with advanced tools for tracking client progress and performance. Fitness apps and wearable devices can monitor metrics such as steps taken, calories burned, distance covered, and even heart rate during workouts. Trainers can use this data to assess clients' progress, identify areas of improvement, and make necessary adjustments to their training programs. Performance tracking also allows clients to visually see their progress, which further enhances motivation and adherence to their fitness goals.

5. Nutrition Monitoring:

Technology plays a significant role in nutrition monitoring, which is a crucial aspect of personal training. Nutrition tracking apps and software can help clients keep a record of their daily food intake and monitor macronutrient distribution. Trainers can use this information to provide nutritional guidance, identify any deficiencies or imbalances, and create personalized meal plans. Integration of technology simplifies the process of tracking and assessing nutritional habits, helping clients establish healthier eating patterns.

6. Virtual Training Sessions:

Technology enables personal trainers to conduct virtual training sessions, expanding their reach and accessibility. Video conferencing platforms allow trainers to guide clients through workouts in real-time, providing instructions, demonstrating exercises, and correcting form. Virtual training sessions can be especially beneficial for clients who have busy schedules, travel frequently, or live in remote locations. Trainers can maintain the accountability and effectiveness of in-person training sessions through virtual platforms.

7. Exercise Libraries and Demonstrations:

Personal training tools and technology offer access to vast exercise libraries and demonstrations. Trainers can utilize fitness apps, websites, and videos to demonstrate proper exercise technique and create comprehensive exercise libraries for their clients. This ensures that clients have visual guidance on how to perform exercises correctly and reduces the risk of injury. Exercise libraries also provide variety and options for trainers to design diverse and engaging workouts.

8. Motivation and Accountability:

Technology can play a crucial role in keeping clients motivated and accountable. Fitness tracking devices and apps provide real-time feedback, reminders, and goals, which keep clients engaged and focused on their progress. Trainers can also use social media platforms or online communities to create a support network for clients, fostering motivation and healthy competition. The integration of technology enhances the overall client experience and helps maintain adherence to the training program.

9. Data Analysis and Insights:

The use of personal training tools and technology generates a wealth of data that can be analyzed to gain valuable insights. Trainers can interpret trends and patterns in clients' data, such as workout intensity, sleep quality, or nutritional habits, to optimize training programs and make data-driven decisions. This data analysis allows for continuous improvement, enabling trainers to refine their approach and provide even better results for their clients.

10. Continuous Learning and Professional Development: Technology provides personal trainers with opportunities for continuous learning and professional development. There are numerous online courses, webinars, and educational resources available that trainers can access to expand their knowledge and stay up-to-date with the latest industry trends. Personal training software and tools also provide trainers with analytics and reports that help them assess their own performance and identify areas for improvement.

6.2 Fitness Tracking Apps and Devices

In the ever-evolving world of personal training, fitness tracking apps and devices have become invaluable tools for both personal trainers and clients. These innovative technologies provide real-time monitoring and analysis of various fitness metrics, enhancing the effectiveness and accountability of personal training programs. Fitness tracking apps and devices offer a range of features, from activity tracking to heart rate monitoring, that can greatly benefit the business of personal training. Here are some key advantages of incorporating fitness tracking apps and devices into personal training:

1. Activity Tracking:

Fitness tracking apps and devices excel at monitoring and tracking various activities throughout the day. From steps taken to distance covered, these tools provide clients with a comprehensive overview of their daily activity levels. This data helps personal trainers understand their clients' baseline activity levels and make necessary adjustments to their training programs to meet individual goals. Activity tracking also promotes accountability and motivation for clients to engage in regular physical activity.

2. Heart Rate Monitoring:

Heart rate monitoring is a crucial aspect of personal training, as it provides insights into intensity levels during workouts. Many fitness tracking apps and devices employ optical sensors or chest straps to accurately measure heart rate. Trainers can analyze this data to ensure that clients are exercising within their target heart rate zones, optimizing the effectiveness of their workouts. Heart rate monitoring also helps prevent overexertion and minimizes the risk of injury.

3. Sleep Tracking:

Quality sleep is essential for recovery and overall well-being. Fitness tracking apps and devices often include sleep tracking features that monitor the duration and quality of sleep. Trainers can access this information to assess clients' sleep patterns and make necessary recommendations for improving sleep quality. Adequate sleep enhances recovery, energy levels, and overall performance, making it an important aspect of personal training.

4. Nutrition Tracking:

Nutrition plays a crucial role in achieving fitness goals, and fitness tracking apps often include features to monitor food intake. Clients can log their meals, track macronutrient distribution, and monitor calorie consumption using these apps. Personal trainers can then access this data to provide nutritional guidance, identify any deficiencies, and help clients make healthier food choices. Nutrition tracking empowers clients to take control of their dietary habits and supports their overall fitness journey.

5. GPS Tracking:

Many fitness tracking apps and devices include GPS functionality, allowing clients to track their outdoor activities such as running or cycling. GPS tracking provides valuable data on distance, pace, and elevation, enabling trainers to monitor progress and design more accurate training programs. Trainers can analyze this data to identify areas for improvement, set realistic goals, and ensure clients are pushing themselves appropriately.

6. Goal Setting and Progress Tracking:

Fitness tracking apps and devices offer features for setting goals and tracking progress. Clients can set specific targets, such as weight loss, muscle gain, or running distance, and monitor their progress towards these goals. Personal trainers can provide guidance and support in setting realistic goals and help clients stay motivated throughout their fitness journey. Progress tracking also allows trainers to assess the effectiveness of the training program and make any necessary adjustments.

7. Data Analysis and Insights:

One of the primary advantages of fitness tracking apps and devices is the data they generate. Trainers can access detailed reports and analytics, such as workout summaries, sleep patterns, and heart rate zones, which provide valuable insights into clients' overall fitness and progress. Analyzing this data enables trainers to identify trends, optimize training programs, and make data-driven decisions to enhance client outcomes.

8. Remote Monitoring and Communication:

Fitness tracking apps and devices allow for remote monitoring and communication between personal trainers and clients. Trainers can access clients' data and provide feedback, guidance, and support through the app or device. This remote monitoring capability helps trainers stay connected with clients and ensures that they are consistently progressing towards their goals. It also allows trainers to offer suggestions and modifications in real-time, further enhancing the client experience.

9. Motivation and Accountability:

Fitness tracking apps and devices are excellent motivators, as they provide clients with tangible evidence of their progress. Seeing improvements in activity levels, heart rate, or sleep quality can immensely boost a client's motivation and commitment to their training program. Trainers can leverage this feature to foster accountability and encourage clients to maintain consistency and adherence to their fitness goals.

10. Integration with Personal Training Programs:

Fitness tracking apps and devices often integrate seamlessly with personal training programs, allowing trainers to incorporate client data directly into their training plans. This integration streamlines the monitoring and analysis process, enabling trainers to provide personalized and data-driven recommendations to their clients. It also enhances the overall client experience by creating a holistic approach to personal training.

6.3 Virtual Training and Online Platforms

The rise of virtual training and online platforms has transformed the landscape of personal training, offering new opportunities for trainers and clients alike. With advancements in technology, personal trainers can now reach a broader audience and provide personalized training programs through virtual training sessions and online platforms. This innovative approach to personal training brings several advantages and benefits for both trainers and clients. Here are key reasons why virtual training and online platforms are valuable personal training tools:

1. Accessibility and Convenience:

Virtual training and online platforms provide clients with unparalleled accessibility and convenience. Geographical barriers are eliminated, allowing clients to train with their desired personal trainer regardless of their physical location. Clients can access their workouts, and training materials, and communicate with their trainer anytime, anywhere through online platforms. This flexibility and convenience make it easier for clients to fit training sessions into their busy schedules, leading to improved adherence and consistency.

2. Cost-Effectiveness:

Virtual training and online platforms often offer more cost-effective options compared to in-person training. Clients can save on travel expenses and gym memberships, as virtual training sessions can be conducted from the comfort of their own homes. Personal trainers can also benefit from this cost-effectiveness, as they can reach a larger client base without the need for a physical gym space. This allows trainers to offer their services at a more affordable rate, making personal training more accessible to a wider range of individuals.

3. Personalized Training:

Virtual training and online platforms enable personal trainers to provide highly personalized training programs. Trainers can use video conferencing platforms to guide clients through workouts in real-time, offering feedback and correcting form. By leveraging technology, trainers can maintain the same level of individualized attention and instruction as in-person training sessions. They can also tailor training programs based on clients' goals, fitness levels, and equipment availability, ensuring that clients receive the personalized attention they need.

4. Variety of Workout Options:

Virtual training and online platforms offer a wide variety of workout options to cater to different client preferences and goals. Trainers can design and deliver diverse workouts using bodyweight exercises, minimal equipment, or equipment that clients have access to at home. Online platforms often provide extensive exercise libraries and pre-recorded workout sessions, allowing clients to choose from a range of workouts that suit their interests and fitness levels. The variety of workout options enhances client engagement and prevents boredom, leading to increased motivation and adherence.

5. Real-Time Feedback and Accountability:

Through virtual training sessions, personal trainers can provide real-time feedback to clients, ensuring that exercises are performed correctly and safely. Trainers can closely observe and correct form, offer modifications or progressions, and provide encouragement, just as they would in an in-person setting. This immediate feedback enhances client learning and performance, fostering a sense of accountability and motivation. Additionally, trainers can utilize online tracking tools and progress monitoring features to hold clients accountable and track their progress towards their goals.

6. Flexibility in Scheduling:

Virtual training and online platforms offer flexibility in scheduling for both trainers and clients. Trainers can accommodate clients in different time zones or clients with varying schedules. Clients can also have greater choices in terms of training times, allowing them to select sessions that best fit their daily routines. This flexibility in scheduling reduces barriers to training and makes personal training more accessible to individuals with demanding lifestyles or irregular work hours.

7. Increased Client Engagement:

Virtual training and online platforms offer enhanced opportunities for client engagement. Trainers can use various online tools such as chat features, video demonstrations, and progress tracking platforms to keep clients engaged and motivated. Trainers can also create online communities or group training sessions, fostering a supportive environment where clients can interact with one another, share experiences, and form connections. This increased engagement improves client satisfaction and helps establish long-term relationships between trainers and clients.

8. Continuity in Training:

Virtual training and online platforms provide trainers and clients the ability to continue training during unforeseen circumstances or disruptions. Inclement weather, travel restrictions, or personal commitments no longer pose significant obstacles to training. Clients can maintain their training routines and progress towards their goals by simply logging into the online platform or joining a virtual training session. This continuity in training ensures that clients stay motivated and focused on their fitness journey, even in challenging circumstances.

9. Continuing Education and Support:

Virtual training and online platforms offer trainers abundant opportunities for continuing education and support.

Trainers can attend webinars, online workshops, and educational programs to expand their knowledge and stay updated with industry trends. Online platforms often provide resources, forums, and networking opportunities that facilitate knowledge sharing and collaboration among trainers. This continuous learning enables trainers to deliver the latest and most effective training techniques to their clients, ensuring high-quality services.

10. Enhanced Trainer Professionalism and Branding:

Embracing virtual training and online platforms can enhance a personal trainer's professionalism and branding. By offering online training services, trainers demonstrate their adaptability and willingness to meet the evolving needs of their clients. Establishing a strong online presence also allows trainers to showcase their expertise, testimonials, and client success stories. Building a reputable online brand not only attracts new clients but also helps trainers differentiate themselves in a crowded market, ultimately leading to business growth and success.

Chapter seven

Marketing and Growing Your Personal Training Business

7.1 Branding and Positioning

In the competitive market of personal training, building a strong brand and positioning yourself effectively can make all the difference in attracting and retaining clients. Branding and positioning strategies are essential for marketing and growing your personal training business. By establishing a distinct brand identity and positioning yourself as an expert in your niche, you can stand out from the competition, attract your ideal clients, and build a successful and thriving business. Here are key factors to consider when it comes to branding and positioning for marketing and growing your personal training business:

1. Define Your Brand Identity:

Branding starts with defining your brand identity, which encompasses your mission, values, personality, and unique selling proposition (USP). Your brand identity is what sets you apart from other personal trainers and resonates with your target audience. Consider what values and beliefs drive your approach to personal training and how you want to be perceived by clients. Develop a compelling USP that communicates the benefits and value you provide to clients. Your brand identity will serve as the foundation for all your marketing efforts and client interactions.

2. Identify Your Target Audience:

To effectively market and grow your personal training business, it is crucial to identify your target audience. Understand who your ideal clients are, their demographic profiles, motivations, goals, and pain points. This knowledge will help you tailor your marketing messages and services to meet their specific needs and desires. Identifying your target audience allows you to create content and marketing campaigns that resonate with them, increasing the chances of attracting and retaining clients who are the right fit for your services.

3. Develop a Consistent Visual Brand:

Consistency in your visual brand is essential for creating recognition and conveying professionalism. Design a logo, choose a color palette, and select fonts that align with your brand identity. Use these visual elements consistently across all your marketing materials, including your website, social media profiles, email newsletters, and printed materials. A visually consistent brand creates a cohesive and professional image, making it easier for clients to recognize and remember your personal training business.

4. Craft a Compelling Brand Story:

A compelling brand story helps you connect with your audience on an emotional level and establishes a genuine connection. Share your personal journey, experiences, and achievements as a personal trainer. Your brand story should demonstrate your expertise, authenticity, and the transformations you have helped clients achieve. Use storytelling techniques to engage your audience and make them feel inspired and motivated to work with you. A strong brand story can differentiate you from competitors and build trust with potential clients.

5. Position Yourself as an Expert:

Positioning yourself as an expert in your niche is vital for attracting clients and establishing credibility. Identify your area of expertise or specialization, and focus your marketing efforts on showcasing your knowledge and skills in that area. Share valuable content, tips, and insights on your website, blog, social media channels, and through guest contributions on relevant platforms. Consistently provide evidence of your expertise, such as certifications, testimonials, case studies, and success stories. By positioning yourself as an expert, you become the go-to personal trainer in your niche, attracting clients who are seeking specialized services.

6. Provide Exceptional Client Experiences:

Delivering exceptional client experiences is crucial for building a positive reputation and promoting word-of-mouth referrals. Focus on providing personalized attention, exceptional customer service, and tailored training programs that address the specific needs and goals of each client. Go above and beyond to exceed their expectations, showing them that you genuinely care about their progress and well-being. By consistently delivering exceptional client experiences, you can build a loyal client base and generate positive reviews and testimonials that contribute to your brand's reputation and growth.

7. Leverage Social Media and Online Platforms:

In today's digital age, leveraging social media and online platforms is essential for marketing and growing your personal training business. Establish a strong online presence by creating professional profiles on popular social media platforms like Facebook, Instagram, LinkedIn, and YouTube. Share valuable content, engage with your audience, and showcase your expertise through informative posts, videos, and live sessions. Utilize online platforms and communities related to health, fitness, and wellness to further expand your reach and visibility. By consistently sharing valuable content and building relationships online, you can attract and retain clients and position yourself as a trusted authority in the personal training industry.

8. Collaborate and Network with Industry Professionals: Collaborating and networking with other industry professionals can significantly contribute to the growth of your personal training business. Form partnerships with local gyms, wellness centers, and other professionals in related fields, such as nutritionists, physical therapists, and sports coaches. Offer complementary services, cross-promote each other, and participate in events or workshops together. Collaborating and networking not only expands your client base but also strengthens your professional network and enhances your credibility and visibility in the industry.

9. Collect and Utilize Client Testimonials:

Client testimonials are powerful tools for establishing credibility, trust, and social proof. Request feedback and testimonials from satisfied clients and showcase them prominently on your website and marketing materials. Testimonials provide potential clients with insight into the positive experiences others have had with your services, increasing their confidence in your abilities. Encourage clients to share their success stories on social media platforms or review websites, further boosting your brand's reputation and attracting more clients.

10. Continuously Monitor and Adapt Your Branding Strategy:

Finally, it is essential to continuously monitor and adapt your branding strategy to stay relevant and competitive. Regularly evaluate your marketing efforts, track the effectiveness of different channels, and listen to client feedback. Be open to making adjustments to your brand positioning, messaging, or target audience if necessary. Stay informed about industry trends, changes, and emerging opportunities, and be proactive in evolving your branding strategy to stay ahead of the competition.

7.2 Marketing Strategies for Acquiring Clients

As a personal trainer, acquiring new clients is essential for growing your business and increasing your revenue. To effectively acquire clients, you need to implement proven marketing strategies that attract and convert potential customers into loyal clients. In this section, we will explore various marketing strategies that can help you acquire clients and grow your personal training business.

1. Define Your Target Market:

Before implementing any marketing strategies, it is crucial to have a clear understanding of your target market. Identify the specific demographics and characteristics of the individuals you want to attract as clients. Consider factors such as age, gender, location, fitness goals, and income level. By understanding your target market, you can tailor your marketing efforts to reach the right audience and maximize your chances of acquiring new clients.

2. Develop a Strong Online Presence:

In today's digital age, having a strong online presence is vital for marketing your personal training business. Create a professional website that showcases your services, qualifications, and client success stories. Optimize your website for search engines to increase your visibility online. Utilize social media platforms such as Facebook, Instagram, and YouTube to share valuable content, engage with your audience, and promote your services. Building a strong online presence can help you reach a wider audience and attract potential clients to your business.

3. Content Marketing:

Content marketing is an effective strategy for attracting potential clients and building credibility in the personal training industry. Create valuable and informative content that addresses the needs and concerns of your target audience. This could include blog posts, videos, podcasts, and infographics. Share this content on your website, social media platforms, and other relevant channels. By consistently providing valuable content, you position yourself as an expert in your field and attract potential clients who are seeking your knowledge and expertise.

4. Use Social Media Advertising:

Social media advertising is a powerful tool for reaching a large audience and driving traffic to your personal training business. Platforms like Facebook and Instagram offer advanced targeting features that allow you to reach individuals who match your target market criteria. Consider running targeted ads that highlight your unique selling points, such as certifications, success stories, and specialized services. Social media advertising can help you generate leads and convert them into paying clients.

5. Offer Free Trials or Consultations:

Offering free trials or consultations is an effective way to demonstrate the value of your services to potential clients. Allow individuals to experience your training firsthand, giving them a taste of what they can expect if they become paying clients. This helps build trust and showcases your expertise. During the trial or consultation, focus on providing exceptional service and addressing their specific goals and concerns. This personal touch can significantly increase the likelihood of converting them into paying clients.

6. Referral Programs:

Word-of-mouth marketing is one of the most powerful forms of advertising. Encourage your existing clients to refer their friends, family, and coworkers to your personal training business. Offer incentives, such as discounts or free training sessions, to clients who refer new customers. The referral program not only helps you acquire new clients but also strengthens relationships with your existing ones. Providing excellent service and results will encourage satisfied clients to refer others to your business.

7. Local Partnerships:

Partnering with local businesses and organizations can be a mutually beneficial marketing strategy. Look for opportunities to collaborate with gyms, sports clubs, wellness centers, and other businesses in your area. Offer special promotions or discounts to their members and clients, and in return, they can promote your services to their audience. By tapping into their existing customer base, you can increase brand visibility and acquire new clients who are already interested in fitness and wellness.

8. Host Workshops or Seminars:

Hosting workshops or seminars is an excellent way to showcase your expertise and attract potential clients. Choose topics that are relevant to your target audience's interests and concerns. For example, you could host a seminar on nutrition, weight loss, or injury prevention. Provide valuable information and actionable tips during these events. This positions you as an authority in your field and allows potential clients to see the value you can provide. Collect contact information from participants and follow up with personalized offers to convert them into paying clients.

9. Online Advertising:

In addition to social media advertising, consider utilizing other online advertising platforms to promote your personal training business. Google Ads and display advertising can help you reach individuals who are actively searching for fitness-related services. Use strategic keywords and compelling ad copy to attract potential clients to your website or landing page. Online advertising allows you to target specific geographic locations and demographics, maximizing your chances of acquiring new clients.

10. Build Relationships:

Building strong relationships in the fitness and wellness community is essential for acquiring new clients. Attend industry events, conferences, and trade shows to connect with other professionals and potential clients. Contribute to online forums and communities related to fitness and wellness. Engage with your audience on social media, responding to comments and messages promptly. By building relationships with others in your industry and with potential clients, you can increase your visibility and attract new clients through referrals and recommendations.

11. Track and Analyze Results:

To optimize your marketing efforts, it is crucial to track and analyze results. Utilize tools like Google Analytics to monitor website traffic, conversion rates, and other key metrics. Track the sources of your client acquisitions to determine which marketing strategies are most effective. Analyze data regularly and make adjustments to your marketing plan accordingly. By understanding what works and what doesn't, you can refine your marketing strategies and maximize your return on investment.

7.3 Building Clientele and Retention Techniques

Building a strong clientele and retaining clients is crucial for the success and growth of your personal training business. While acquiring new clients is important, it is equally essential to focus on customer retention and building long-term relationships with your clients. In this section, we will explore effective techniques for building your clientele and strategies for retaining clients in the personal training industry.

1. Exceptional Customer Service:

Providing exceptional customer service is the foundation for building and retaining clients in any business, and personal training is no exception. Always prioritize your clients' needs and go above and beyond to ensure their satisfaction. Take the time to listen to their goals, concerns, and progress. Tailor your training programs to their individual needs and preferences. Show genuine care and interest in their well-being and progress. By consistently delivering exceptional customer service, you create a positive experience that encourages clients to stay with your business and refer others to you.

2. Personalization and Individual Attention:

One of the key advantages of personal training is the ability to provide personalized attention and guidance to clients. Tailor your training programs to each client's specific goals, fitness level, and preferences. Treat each client as an individual and develop a personalized approach to their training journey. Regularly assess their progress, adjust workouts accordingly, and provide ongoing motivation and support. By providing personalized training and individual attention, you demonstrate your commitment to each client and enhance their overall experience, increasing the likelihood of long-term retention.

3. Goal Setting and Progress Tracking:

Helping clients set specific, measurable, attainable, realistic, and time-bound (SMART) goals is an effective technique for client retention. Work collaboratively with clients to establish short-term and long-term goals that align with their overall fitness objectives. Regularly track and measure their progress using various metrics, such as body measurements, body fat percentage, strength gains, and endurance improvements. Celebrate their achievements and provide ongoing feedback on their progress. By actively tracking and reviewing their progress, you keep clients engaged and motivated, increasing their commitment to your training program.

4. Customized Training Programs:

Offering customized training programs is a powerful retention technique for personal trainers. Design programs that cater to each client's unique needs, preferences, and limitations. Incorporate a variety of exercises, equipment, and training modalities to keep the workouts interesting and challenging. Regularly update and modify the training programs to prevent boredom and ensure continued progress. By providing customized training programs, you keep clients engaged and motivated, reducing the risk of attrition.

5. Communication and Availability:

Maintaining open and regular communication with clients is essential for client retention. Be responsive to their inquiries, concerns, and feedback. Use various communication channels, such as in-person meetings, phone calls, emails, and text messages, to stay connected and provide ongoing support. Consistently check in with clients to gauge their satisfaction, progress, and any challenges they may be facing. This demonstrates your dedication to their success and fosters a sense of trust and loyalty.

6. Building Relationships:

Developing strong relationships with your clients goes beyond the personal training sessions. Take the time to get to know your clients on a personal level, showing genuine interest in their lives outside the gym. Remember details about their families, hobbies, and interests. Celebrate special occasions, such as birthdays and achievements, with personalized gestures. Building meaningful relationships with your clients fosters a sense of belonging and connection, making them more likely to remain loyal to your business.

7. Continuous Education and Professional Development: Continuously investing in your own education and professional development is essential for client retention. Stay up-to-date with the latest industry trends, research, and techniques. Participate in relevant workshops, conferences, and training programs to enhance your knowledge and skills. By continuously improving your expertise, you provide added value to your clients and position yourself as a knowledgeable and experienced trainer. Clients are more likely to stay with a trainer who demonstrates a commitment to ongoing learning and improvement.

8. Rewards and Incentives:

Implementing a rewards and incentives program is an effective strategy for client retention. Offer rewards such as discounts, free sessions, or exclusive merchandise for achieving specific milestones, referring new clients, or staying committed to their training program for a certain duration. Gamify the training experience by setting challenges or competitions with incentives for the winners. The rewards and incentives program not only provides tangible benefits to your clients but also keeps them engaged and motivated on their fitness journey.

9. Community Building:

Creating a sense of community among your clients can significantly contribute to client retention. Organize group training sessions, workshops, or social events where clients can interact and develop relationships with each other. Encourage clients to support and motivate each other, fostering a positive and inclusive training environment. Consider creating an online community or forum where clients can connect, share their experiences, and seek support. By building a sense of community, clients feel a sense of belonging and are more likely to remain committed to your training business.

10. Regular Assessments and Check-ins:
Regularly assessing and reviewing clients' progress is important for client retention. Schedule periodic assessments to track their achievements, reassess their goals, and make necessary adjustments to their training programs. Conduct regular check-ins to ensure client satisfaction and address any concerns or challenges. By demonstrating your ongoing commitment to their progress, you strengthen the client-trainer relationship and create a sense of accountability and support.

11. Client Feedback and Surveys:

Seeking regular client feedback is crucial for understanding their needs, preferences, and satisfaction levels. Implement a system for collecting client feedback, such as surveys or comment cards. Encourage clients to share their opinions, suggestions, and concerns. Actively listen to their feedback and make necessary improvements to your services and programs. By incorporating client feedback into your business practices, you show your clients that their opinions are valued, and you continuously strive to provide an exceptional experience.

12. Client Retention Programs:

Implementing client retention programs can help you proactively reduce attrition and encourage long-term commitment. Offer loyalty discounts or bonuses for clients who renew their training packages or commit to long-term training contracts. Provide exclusive benefits or access to additional services for loyal clients. Design programs that address the specific needs and concerns of your long-term clients, such as specialized workshops or advanced training sessions. By investing in client retention programs, you solidify the loyalty of your existing clientele and increase the likelihood of long-term retention.

Chapter eight

Taking Your Personal Training Business Online

8.1 Benefits and Challenges of Online Training

In recent years, there has been a significant shift towards online platforms for various industries, including the fitness industry. With advances in technology and increased accessibility to the internet, personal trainers have the opportunity to take their businesses online. This transition offers numerous benefits but also presents certain challenges. In this section, we will explore the benefits and challenges of online training for taking your personal training business online.

Benefits of Online Training:

1. Increased Reach and Access: One of the biggest advantages of online training is the ability to reach a wider audience. Without geographical limitations, you can attract clients from different parts of the world, expanding your potential client base exponentially. Online training also provides accessibility to individuals who may have limited access or mobility issues, making fitness training more inclusive.

2. Flexibility and Convenience: Online training offers flexibility for both the trainer and the client. Trainers can set their own schedules and work from anywhere, while clients can choose their preferred training sessions based on their own availability. This flexibility is particularly beneficial for individuals with busy lifestyles or irregular work hours.

3. Cost-Effective: From a business perspective, taking your personal training business online can be more cost-effective compared to maintaining a physical gym or studio. You can save on overhead expenses such as rent, utilities, and equipment maintenance. Additionally, online training enables you to reach and train multiple clients simultaneously, maximizing your earning potential.

4. Personalized Training Programs: Online training allows you to provide personalized training programs to each client efficiently. Through online platforms or applications, you can gather information about clients' goals, fitness levels, and preferences, and create customized training programs tailored to their specific needs. This personalized approach enhances the client experience and increases the chances of achieving their desired results.

5. Convenient Communication and Support: With online training, communication between the trainer and client can occur through various channels, such as video calls, emails, or messaging apps. This provides a convenient and immediate means of support and guidance for clients. Trainers can offer real-time feedback, answer questions, and provide motivation and accountability, even when physically distant.

6. Increased Client Engagement: Online training offers unique opportunities to engage and motivate clients through virtual challenges, online communities, and progress tracking tools. By incorporating gamification and social interactions, you can boost client engagement and long-term adherence to their fitness program.

Challenges of Online Training:

1. Lack of Physical Presence: One of the primary challenges of online training is the absence of physical presence. Trainers are unable to physically observe and correct clients' form, which increases the risk of injury or ineffective workouts. It requires trainers to rely heavily on verbal cues and video demonstrations to guide clients accurately.

2. Technical Difficulties: Online training heavily relies on technology, which means that technical issues can arise, such as poor internet connectivity, video call disruptions, or software glitches. These technical difficulties can interrupt training sessions and hinder smooth communication between the trainer and client.

3. Limited Equipment and Space: Online training may also present challenges regarding equipment

availability and the suitability of clients' training spaces. Clients may have limited access to fitness equipment or may not have enough space to perform certain exercises effectively. Trainers need to be creative in designing workouts that utilize minimal equipment or adapt exercises based on clients' available resources.

4. Self-Motivation and Accountability: Online training requires a high level of self-motivation and accountability from clients. Without the physical presence of a trainer, some individuals may struggle to stay committed and consistent with their training program. Trainers need to devise strategies to keep clients motivated, such as regular check-ins, goal setting, and progress tracking.

5. Privacy and Security Concerns: Online training involves sharing personal information and potentially conducting video calls or sessions in

clients' homes. Trainers need to be mindful of privacy and security concerns to ensure client confidentiality and protect sensitive information. Implementing secure communication tools and establishing clear privacy policies are crucial in maintaining trust and professionalism.

6. Client Education and Knowledge Transfer: Online training requires trainers to find effective ways to educate and transfer knowledge to clients in a remote setting. Trainers must ensure that clients understand proper exercise techniques, training principles, and safety guidelines without the benefit of real-time demonstrations. The use of instructional videos, written resources, and clear communication becomes essential in bridging this gap.

8.2 Creating and Delivering Online Training Programs

With the increasing popularity of online training, personal trainers are looking for ways to transition their businesses online to reach a wider audience and provide more flexibility to their clients. Creating and delivering online training programs requires a different set of skills and tools than traditional in-person training. In this section, we will explore the steps involved in creating and delivering successful online training programs for taking your personal training business online.

Step 1: Define your target audience and goals:

Before creating an online training program, it is essential to define your target audience and their specific fitness goals. Identify what your clients need and what you can offer to help them succeed. Tailor your program to meet their unique needs and preferences. Additionally, establish measurable goals that align with your clients' desired outcomes and track progress.

Step 2: Choose the right platform:

Select a platform that is suitable for delivering your online training program. There are numerous options available, such as video conferencing tools, online fitness platforms, and social media platforms. Consider the features, accessibility, and compatibility of each platform to determine the best fit for your clients' needs.

Step 3: Create a program structure and schedule:

Design a program structure that guides clients systematically towards their fitness goals. Develop a comprehensive training plan, including strength training, cardio workouts, and nutrition recommendations. Create a schedule that accommodates clients' availability and customizes the program based on their fitness level and goals.

Step 4: Utilize multimedia tools for engagement and motivation:

Incorporate multimedia tools into your online training program to increase client engagement and motivation. Utilize instructional videos, animated graphics, and interactive tools such as quizzes, gamification strategies, and virtual challenges. These elements enhance the learning experience and promote client adherence to the program.

Step 5: Incorporate accountability measures:

Accountability is critical in ensuring clients stay on track with their fitness program. Implement accountability measures such as progress tracking, check-ins, and support groups to motivate clients and keep them on track.

Utilize online tools such as video conferencing and mobile apps to communicate with clients and offer real-time feedback.

Step 6: Promote and market your program:

Promote your online training program to attract potential clients and showcase your expertise. Utilize social media platforms, blogs, and email marketing campaigns to increase visibility and target your ideal client demographic. Offer free trials and discounts to encourage sign-ups and cultivate client loyalty.

Step 7: Continuously review and improve:

Regularly review and improve your online training program to provide the best possible experience for your clients. Seek feedback from clients, analyze program data, and incorporate new industry trends or research. Continual improvement allows you to deliver a relevant and effective program and attract and retain clients.

8.3 Online Marketing and Client Acquisition

Taking your personal training business online opens up limitless possibilities to reach a wider audience and expand your client base. However, in order to be successful, it is essential to have a well-thought-out online marketing strategy to attract and acquire clients. In this section, we will explore effective online marketing techniques to help you grow your personal training business online.

1. Define your target audience:

To create an effective online marketing strategy, it is crucial to define your target audience. Consider factors such as age, gender, location, fitness goals, and preferences. By understanding your target audience's needs and desires, you can tailor your marketing messages and tactics to resonate with them.

2. Create a compelling website:

Your website serves as the virtual storefront for your personal training business. Make sure it is visually appealing, user-friendly, and informative. Include relevant information about your services, credentials, and testimonials. Optimize your website for search engines to increase your visibility in online searches.

3. Develop a strong brand identity:

Create a strong brand identity that aligns with your target audience and differentiates you from competitors. Choose a memorable logo, color scheme, and brand voice. Consistently incorporate your brand elements into your website, social media profiles, and marketing materials to establish brand recognition.

4. Leverage social media platforms:

Social media platforms are powerful tools for promoting your personal training business online. Create engaging and informative content on platforms relevant to your target audience, such as Facebook, Instagram, and LinkedIn. Use a mix of images, videos, and written content to showcase your expertise and attract potential clients. Engage with your audience by responding to comments and messages promptly.

5. Utilize search engine optimization (SEO):

Implementing SEO techniques can improve your website's visibility and ranking in search engine results. Identify relevant keywords related to personal training and optimize your website's content, meta tags, and headers accordingly. Regularly create high-quality and relevant content such as blog posts, videos, and tutorials to keep your website up-to-date.

6. Offer valuable content and resources:

Provide valuable content and resources to your audience to establish yourself as an authoritative figure in the industry. Create informative blog posts, workout videos, nutrition guides, and downloadable resources. Offering free content not only attracts potential clients but also establishes trust and credibility.

7. Implement email marketing campaigns:

Develop an email marketing strategy to nurture leads and engage with your existing clients. Offer sign-ups for newsletters or free resources on your website to capture email addresses. Send regular emails with training tips, success stories, and exclusive offers. Personalize your emails to make them relevant and valuable to each recipient.

8. Collaborate with influencers and partners:

Partnering with influencers, fitness bloggers, or other professionals in complementary industries can help amplify your online presence. Collaborate with them for cross-promotion, guest blogging, or joint online events. Leveraging their audience can introduce your personal training business to a wider network of potential clients.

9. Offer incentives and referrals:

Encourage your existing clients to refer their friends and family to your online training programs by offering incentives. Provide discounts or exclusive services to those who refer new clients. Word-of-mouth referrals can be one of the most effective ways to acquire new clients and grow your business.

10. Track and analyze your marketing efforts:

Regularly track and analyze your online marketing campaigns to understand what is working and what needs improvement. Monitor website traffic, email open rates, social media engagement, and conversion rates. Use this data to refine your marketing strategy and allocate resources effectively.

Conclusion

In conclusion, the business of personal training plays a vital role in helping clients achieve their fitness goals. Whether it's through in-person sessions or taking the business online, personal trainers have the ability to make a significant impact on people's lives.

By providing personalized workout plans, nutrition guidance, and motivation, personal trainers ensure that clients receive the support they need to overcome challenges and make progress towards their fitness goals. They serve as mentors, educators, and cheerleaders, empowering clients to push their limits and become the best version of themselves.

Taking the personal training business online opens up new opportunities to reach a broader audience and provide flexible training options. Online platforms enable trainers to deliver effective workout programs, provide real-time feedback, and foster a sense of community and accountability among clients.

Furthermore, effective online marketing strategies are crucial for acquiring and retaining clients. By defining target audiences, creating strong branding, and utilizing social media, SEO, and email marketing, personal trainers can effectively promote their services and connect with potential clients.

In the rapidly evolving fitness industry, personal trainers must be adaptable and continually improve their skills and knowledge. Staying updated with the latest trends and research allows trainers to offer innovative and evidence-based training methods, enhancing the effectiveness of their programs.

Ultimately, the business of personal training goes beyond physical transformation. Personal trainers have the privilege of not only helping clients achieve their fitness goals but also positively impacting their overall well-being, confidence, and mindset. By providing the support, encouragement, and guidance needed for clients to succeed, personal trainers play a crucial role in helping individuals lead healthier and happier lives.

So, whether you're considering starting a personal training business, expanding your services online, or seeking a personal trainer to help you on your fitness journey, remember the immense value that personal trainers bring in helping individuals achieve their fitness goals.